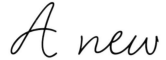 

GW00418636

Contents

Text by Sara Burford.

This edition published in 2008 by L&K Designs.
© L&K Designs 2008
PRINTED IN CHINA

Publishers Disclaimer

The recipes contained in this book are passed on in good faith but the publisher cannot be held responsible for any adverse results. Please be aware that certain recipes may contain nuts.

It is also recommended that you consult your doctor before embarking on any fitness regime or eating programme.

A New You

Investing well-spent time and energy in keeping ourselves fit, healthy and happy on both the inside and the outside, is our finest ally in looking and feeling great – and a well deserved expression of self-care and positive self-image.

Inner and outer beauty is attainable by all, regardless of age, size, shape or style – and it doesn't have to come out of a jar, over a counter or in outlandishly expensive treatments.

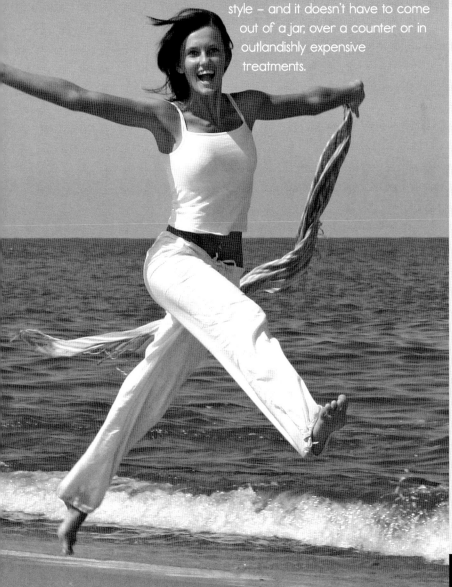

A New You is a simply worded, easy to use guide in achieving inner calm, improved health, enhanced physical energy and sparkling radiance!

Complimented perfectly by creative and handy fashion and beauty tips to optimise your natural looks and personal style.

Combining tips on relaxation and stress relief, energy boosting ideas and exercises with healthy eating 'superfoods', you can't fail to give your mind and body a welcome replenishment of nutrition, vitality and a tranquil sense of wellbeing.

Fabulous tips and remedies for skin and hair care, timeless fashion "Do's and Don'ts" and must-have 5-minute beauty tips will polish off your new found "Joie de vivre" and benefit you further by boosting your confidence and releasing that uber-stylish, self-assured and relaxed New You...

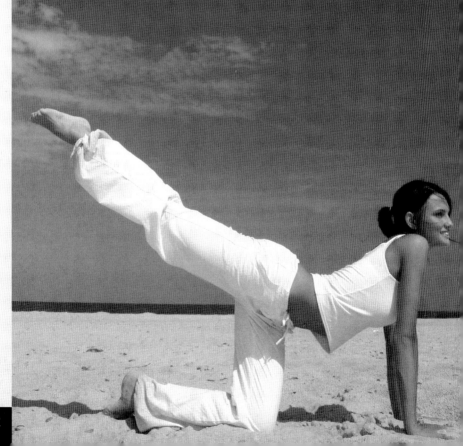

One of the easiest ways to make a change to your well-being is to plan "you-time" in which to relax and unwind. Relaxing calms anxiety and helps your mind and body recover from the everyday hustle and bustle, which can cause stress. Music, a long soak in the bath, or a walk in the park are great ways to relax.

Regularly using a relaxation technique is an easy and effective way to relieve stress and achieve a deeper sense of calm and wellbeing, for both mind and body.

The practice of relaxation techniques can improve how you physically and emotionally respond to stress by lowering blood pressure, slowing the heart rate down, reducing muscle tension and other associated ailments such as headaches and feelings of anger and frustration. Regular relaxation increases energy levels, diminishing the unpleasant symptoms of anxiety.

Relaxation technique

Firstly, minimise distractions, such as turning off the TV or radio and unplugging the phone. Give yourself permission to ignore the doorbell and to deal with the next job or chore later. This is valuable 'YOU-time'.

Sit or lie down in a comfortable position, preferably in a quiet place where you won't be disturbed. Close your eyes and begin to breathe slowly and calmly, inhale through your nose and exhale through your mouth. Notice the rhythm and speed of your breath and slow it down if necessary.

Beginning with your feet, tense and simultaneously relax each part of your body, putting enough tension into your muscles to make them tense but not so that they are painful. Working your way up through your legs and torso tense each muscle eventually ending with your face and head.

Whilst tensing and relaxing each part of your body be aware of your breathing and focus upon the warmth and heaviness of your muscles as you let go of all your tension. Affirming thoughts may help to achieve a deeper feeling of relaxation; "I feel calm and quiet. My body is heavy, comfortable and relaxed. I feel at peace".

Empty your mind, pushing any current distractions or worries to the back of your mind - simply let them float away. Sometimes the visualisation of a calm, relaxing place can be helpful such as a scenic view of a sprawling summer meadow or a sandy beach with the waves lapping at the shore.

Stay in this position for about 20 minutes, then take some deep breaths, open your eyes but remain sitting or lying for a few more moments before getting up.

For relaxation techniques to be of optimum use, it is a good idea to make space for them in your everyday life.

Coping with stress

Having a little bit of stress in our lives isn't a negative thing; small amounts of stress serves to mobilise our bodies providing us with the necessary energy and verve to take us through the process of coping with challenges.

However, having too much stress in our lives can lead to a wide range of health problems including, upset stomach, headaches, depression, anxiety attacks, high blood pressure and even conditions as serious as heart disease or strokes.

Stress is a normal part of life and as such we can worsen the symptoms of stress by giving ourselves a hard time for even feeling them in the first place.

So first and foremost, be easy on yourself - self-criticism will only expend unnecessary energy and make an already stressful time harder to deal with.

Stress relieving tips

Be kind to yourself, do something relaxing that you enjoy on a regular basis, such as taking a scenic walk or treating yourself to a candlelit bath whilst listening to your favourite CD.

Alcohol
Don't reach for alcohol in times of stress, it may bring short-term relief but alcohol is a depressant and will inhibit restful sleep, as well as the added strain of having to deal with processing toxins through your system the following day.

Aromatherapy
An ancient Chinese tradition, aromatherapy is based on the healing properties of plant extracts which are bottled as 'essential oils'. The oils are inhaled and circulated through the bloodstream, having an effect on the release of the hormones and emotions of the user. For example, Lavender oil is used to help in relieving stress, tension, mental exhaustion, anxiety and agitation.

Breathing

Be aware of your body and breathing, notice any tension in your muscles and breathe deeply, gently stretching out and relaxing your muscles.

Classes

Invest time and energy in yourself by taking up a class in something you have an interest in, such as pottery or flower arranging, or perhaps learning a different language. Something that isn't overtly challenging or in any way stressful, allowing you to meet new people, relax and enjoy yourself whilst learning a new and interesting skill.

De-clutter

Mess adds to confusion and feelings of powerlessness so de-clutter!

If you are surrounded by clutter and disorganisation be dynamic and have a good clear out and tidy. You will get a sense of satisfaction and feel far more in control.

Diary

Keep a journal – or a stress diary. Some people find that writing down their thoughts and feelings can be extremely helpful, and an effective way of putting their problems in perspective, or in coming up with solutions to solve the problems they are experiencing.

Diet

Eat a balanced diet for a healthy body and mind. When our bodies are nutritionally boosted we possess a greater capacity for dealing with the effects of stress.

Easy on the eye!

Place something you really enjoy looking at in optimum view in your house or room, perhaps fresh flowers, a favourite picture or a treasured ornament.

Exercise

Exercise regularly; physical exercise has great benefits in managing and reducing stress.

Exercise is a fabulous stress buster and you don't have to be a gym dweller or high-impact cardiovascular devotee to reap the benefits from regular exercise. Just 20-30 minutes brisk walking 3 times a week will reduce stress and help aid more restful sleep. This can be either be maintained or increased over time depending on your fitness level and ability.

Exercise relieves stress by allowing the body to release pent-up tension and frustration - relaxing muscles and raising the level of endorphins within the brain, which are our 'feel good' chemicals. Taking regular exercise mobilises our bodies, keeps us in a better state of health and consequently makes us feel good about ourselves. Take up stress relieving relaxing exercise such as Tai Chi or Yoga, which are renowned for their relaxation qualities and techniques. Meditation is another popular method of relaxation and effective stress relief.

Hobbies

Take time out for an enjoyable activity whenever you can, such as playing a sport, taking a trip to the cinema or seeing your favourite band play.

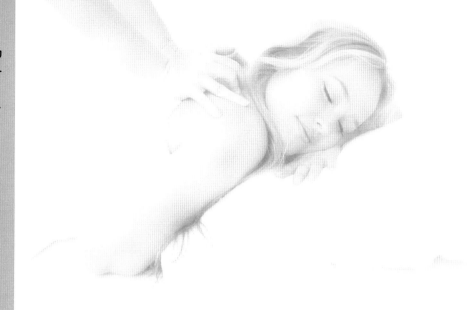

Massage

Massage is one of the oldest forms of health disciplines designed to treat stress and promote relaxation.

A massage performed by a professionally trained masseur can provide deep relaxation by working on tense muscles and physiologically improving circulation.

As muscles start to relax the body and mind naturally follow suit and an enhanced feeling of calm can be achieved.

Meditation

Meditation has become a part of our popular culture and due to its positive and often immediate results, is often recommended by Doctors for reducing stress and pain management.

Meditation involves sitting in a relaxed position, closing your eyes and clearing the mind, focusing upon your breathing, an image, word or sound, which allows you to be distraction-free and completely relaxed.

It is best to set aside between 10-20 minutes of free time in a quiet and private space.

The practice of meditation lowers the heart rate, slows down breathing; thus using oxygen more effectively, and lowers blood pressure.

This process of mind clearing and relaxation is thought to promote feelings of being deeply rested and calm, both during and directly following practice.

There are different forms of meditation available, some schools of thought teach concentration techniques, some relaxation and others a more free form of contemplative techniques.

Music
Listening to music can do wonders to alleviate stress. Choosing to play a familiar and relaxing tune which soothes you can help to deepen breathing, reduce heart rate, lower cortisol levels, (the stress hormone), increase the production of serotonin (the 'happy' hormone), and allow the body to relax.

During a commute we all experience differing levels of stress and research has been undertaken which showed that playing a favourite a piece of music can serve to relieve tension and reduce the risk of road rage!

Positive Mental Attitude
Think Positive – use positive affirmations and repeat them to yourself throughout the day, or put them on post-its dotted around your house.

If you can't think of any, ask someone close to you to write down some of the things that they like about you.

Positive streams of thought can really help to boost your mood and change how you think about yourself.

Reiki

Reiki is a Japanese word, meaning "universal life-force energy" and is used by practitioners as a form of relaxation, stress and pain relief, believed to promote healing on a mental, physical and spiritual level.

Reiki involves the practitioner placing their hands on the recipient and accessing natural vibrational energy – or Reiki energy – and allowing it to flow through to the recipient for the purposes of healing and restoring depleted energy.

Reiki is becoming an increasingly popular method of treatment and incorporates many other alternative and holistic healing rituals, such as crystal therapy, homeopathy, chakra balancing and meditation.

Reiki can produce fast and long-lasting results in dealing with stress, tension, anxiety and related symptoms. It can also help in cases of insomnia and general emotional turmoil and discord.

Reiki can help you acheive a sense of well-being and balance if you are feeling in low spirits or have low energy levels.

Sleep

Get enough sleep – stress will be made worse by tiredness and reduce your ability to think rationally. Too much sugar or caffeine will play a part in preventing restful sleep so be mindful of intake during periods of stress.

Slow down

Walk, talk and eat at a relaxed pace – rushing causes unnecessary stress on your body. Take a short break after meals to allow yourself to relax and aid digestion.

Take time to notice the natural, everyday things in life that we all take for granted like; local scenery, wildlife, the changes of season, feeling the grass beneath your feet, even watching children play. It's amazing how sometimes going back to basics can help us gain some perspective.

Socialise

Spend quality time talking and sharing your life with people that you enjoy being around. After all, no man is an island!

Support

Connect with other people and develop a support network – just talking through personal issues can have a positive effect. Avoid holding in feelings day after day, find a safe and loving place to feel, communicate and embrace them.

Tai Chi

Tai Chi is a Chinese martial art originating in the 13th Century, which aims to improve or maintain good health, condition the body and create a sense of relaxation, fostering a calm and tranquil mind.

As it is practiced in the West today it is more popularly regarded as a moving form of yoga and meditation combined.

Its exercises consist of sequences of smooth, flowing movements, which are performed slowly and gracefully emphasising concentration, relaxation and focusing the body's energy. In addition to its stress relieving benefits Tai Chi promotes improved balance, core stability and correction of poor posture.

Tai Chi is less strenuous than Yoga and as such is considered to be more suitable for all age groups and levels of fitness. The slow motion routines are practiced in parks around the world, most popularly in China.

Yoga

Traditionally an Eastern practice, Yoga has now become one of the most popular forms of physical relaxation and stress relief in the West; building strength, stamina and flexibility whilst increasing energy, improving circulation, boosting the immune system and aiding calmness and natural sleep.

Yoga, meaning 'union' or 'merger', uses movement, breath, stretching, posture and relaxation in order to establish its health benefits.

Daily practice is believed to boost not only flexibility and joint mobility, but also mental clarity and an increased sense of wellbeing.

The popularity of Yoga practice has lead to the formation of widespread classes ranging from complete beginners through to seasoned Yoga practitioners. For further information on classes in your area search your local directories or consult a website such as www.yoga.co.uk

If you can't function in the morning without gallons of coffee and you run out of energy by mid afternoon, then you need to look at simple ways of boosting your energy levels through food and exercise.

Why exercise?

Our bodies are designed to move. When we're not in motion our circulation and energy systems slow down, making us feel lethargic and even less likely to want to mobilise ourselves.

Exercise is a fantastic way of boosting our energy levels and revitalising the whole of our physical and mental wellbeing. We feel less tired, less stressed, happier and healthier. From the very young through to the older generation, exercise is an important activity in our lives and age & fitness appropriate exercise routines can provide much needed 'get-up-and-go' and an enhanced quality of life.

You don't have to jog, run or take part in high impact aerobics should they not suit your sensibilities or physical abilities - although they do have certain health benefits they can also be harsh on joints and muscles and cause wear-and-tear in the long-term. Low impact exercises can be just as beneficial and very enjoyable too!

Exercise – learn to love it!

Many of us hear the word 'exercise' and groan. Exercise is often associated with painful, energy-sapping activities which drain our bank-accounts through well intentioned, but ultimately severely underutilised gym memberships. Consequently, we often end up blocking our willingness to go anywhere near anything remotely looking, or sounding, like an activity which might need some form of physical exertion.

So choosing exercise that we can enjoy is important, as is how we program ourselves to think about exercise. If we think negatively, we will see exercise negatively. So try some more positive thoughts such as "It feels really good to exercise", "I love going out for a long walk in the morning" or "I really enjoy my dancing class".

The more you can think positively and program yourself to enjoy exercise, the easier it will be to overcome those negative thought patterns.

Aqua aerobics

This is the performance of aerobic exercise in shallow water such as a swimming pool. One of the many benefits of performing aerobics in the water is that the water provides support for the body which reduces the risk of muscle or joint injury and because the exercises are usually performed in chest or waist-deep water, you do not have to be a swimmer to participate. Water-related exercise increases cardio-vascular fitness, as well as improving overall strength.

Aqua aerobic workouts usually combine a variety of different techniques, mainly taken from land aerobics. The workout also may incorporate special water devices that can be used in the water to aid in resistance or flotation.

As water provides more resistance than air, in general aqua aerobics will expend more energy than many land-based activities. An aerobic water exercise of around 30 minutes will help burn about 300 calories.

Breathing exercise

Most of us take our breathing for granted, but without sufficient respiration our bodies become tired and sluggish, causing us to suffer from lack of concentration and decreased response times. Just 5-10 minutes of breathing exercises daily increases our body's oxygen levels, improving clarity and alertness and working wonders on our energy levels.

Choose a comfortable position, sitting or lying down. Straighten your back with shoulders not tense but very slightly angled forward, and your chest slightly caved in. Align your head with your spine.

Inhale slowly and evenly through your nose, breathing in deeply by pulling upward the diaphragm muscle which is situated just below your ribcage. Allow your lungs to expand outwards within in your chest cavity and imagine that you are filling your whole abdomen with air.

Pause for a moment and then slowly exhale through your nose, whilst letting your abdomen and chest flatten out – do not force this movement, keep it gentle and even.

Pause for a few seconds and repeat the cycle again for between 5-10 minutes.

Cycling

Cycling is an enjoyable form of low-impact aerobic exercise with many health benefits, including weight loss, improved overall strength and muscle tone, enhanced stamina and coordination, lowered risk of heart attack and stress reduction.

As well as being great exercise which can be enjoyed with family and friends, cycling is also a practical mode of transport!

For safety and security, always wear a helmet and ensure that your clothing is visible in poor light. Inform someone of your intended journey and approximate arrival or return time.

Dancing

Experts say that dancing burns calories, boosts energy, improves circulation and tones muscle leadijng to increased strength, endurance and flexibility. In fact, dancing can burn just as many calories as other, more "traditional" exercises and in addition, dancing relieves tension and stress, improves your mood and serves as an outlet for your creativity. Dancing also is convenient and you don't need any expensive equipment - all you need is your body, some music and the willingness to have fun. Many local YMCAs, health clubs and even gyms offer classes in different dance techniques from modern to jazz, salsa to waltz if you'd like to try something a little different, but the great thing about dancing is that you can also do it in the comfort of your own room. Movie to the music and practice good health and fitness!

Family fun

Exercise is a fun way to spend time together as a family, as well as being an excellent way to keep fit and encourage younger family members to invest in a healthy way of living. Ideas for activities could include rollerblading, a friendly ballgame competition, cycling, swimming, hill-walking, family-friendly assault-courses, choosing an activity oriented holiday such as skiing or sailing, and any local sports, charity fun-runs or keep-fit activities which can be done as a group.

Local classes

Attending a local exercise or fitness class has probably never been easier. There are many different types of class available within communities; at leisure facilities, schools and colleges, local community halls and function rooms. Choices may include aerobics, spinning, yoga, tai chi, aqua-aerobics, pilates, martial arts and dancing. Many classes can be attended at beginner's level through to advanced level, depending on personal ability and interest.

Your local council should be able to provide you with listings of leisure facilities and classes within your area.

Running

Running - you either love it or you hate it; but the health and well-being benefits of running should outweigh the hatred! One of the most common reasons that peope run is to lose weight or get fit, and then to maintain a healthy lifestyle. Some even use running as a way of expanding their social circle by meeting other people to train with or to compete against.

Running also prevents muscle and bone loss that occurs naturally with old age. Running may also help fight disease; it certainly helps to strengthen your heart and whole cardio-vascular system. These are just a few of the health benefits one earns from running.

There are also numerous proven psychological benefits to running as it can help build confidence in all ages of people. Going for a jog can reduce your stress level drastically - and of course, endorphins are the body's natural antidepressant.

It is though easy to strain muscles and suffer other injuries whilst running, so it is important that before undertaking any training programme you discuss this with a doctor or fitness professional and ask their advice about a regime best suited to your abilities.

It will also be necessary to purchase appropriate clothing and in particular shoes so as to ensure that your joints are provided with adequate cushioning when pounding the pavement!

Swimming

Swimming is one of the all-round most beneficial exercises we can undertake, working all the major muscles and massaging the internal organs in the process. As the density of the human body is similar to that of the water, the body is supported within the water and therefore less stress is placed upon joints and bones.

Swimming on a regular basis builds stamina, muscle strength and tone and improves cardio-vascular fitness. It is also proven to promote relaxation and aid stress relief.

Walking

One of the most accessible forms of exercise is walking. The beauty of which lies in its ease and flexibility. Walking can be done alone, in a group, indoors, outdoors - it can be fitted in between break-times at work, leisure time in the evenings or weekends, or even as a regular morning ritual.

Improving the oxygen capacity of the lungs and heart, walking briskly for 20-30 minutes 3-4 times a week has an invigorating effect on energy levels and circulation. To continue improving the benefits of walking, increase the pace and duration over time.

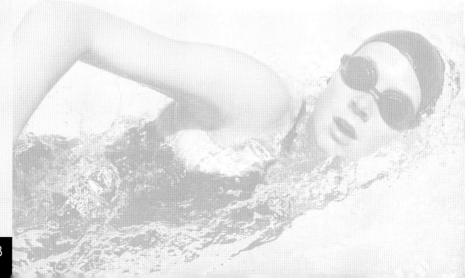

Food – your body's fuel

Following that sugar-filled or fat-laden lunch, how many of us have wanted a mid-afternoon snooze during that all-important meeting, or when we've needed our wits about us to take care of our boundlessly energised children?

Fast, sugary and processed foods serve as quick fixes when we're hungry, but are false energy-economy in the long run.

Just as we fuel our engines to ensure our vehicles run smoothly for a required distance, our bodies need the right type and quantity of fuel to keep us going too.

Eating the wrong types of food, or even too much or too little, can make us feel and look tired and sluggish and have an unfavourable affect on our mental agility and performance.

What we choose to put into our bodies truly does reflect in how we present ourselves and perform.

So how can we energise our bodies with what we eat?

Friendly foods

Foods high in fat, sugar and salt are all known to have an adverse affect on our physical and mental functioning; playing havoc with our energy levels and leaving us often feeling heavy, bloated, lackluster and unhappy with ourselves.

A well-balanced diet enriched with vegetables, green, fruits, vegetable salads, sprouting pulses and grains, nuts and seeds, oily fish, poultry and some dairy produce should see you to a healthier, more invigorated way of feeling and living.

Don't skip meals, By missing any daily meal our bodies are likely to feel more tired and energy-zapped by the end of the day.

Breakfast – an important start

Breakfast is often a meal that we don't have time for in our ever increasingly hectic modern lives. But research has shown that eating a healthy breakfast is vital for energy, concentration and alertness.

In addition to a more energised start to the day, eating breakfast helps to control weight by preventing panic-eating the wrong types of foods, as well as too much food during the day.

In order to gain maximum benefit from the first meal of the day reduce the amount of fried and fatty foods in your diet, as these are linked to low energy levels, and choose instead complex-carbohydrates and protein for sustained energy. Suggestions for combinations could be:-

Plain fat-free yoghurt with reduced-sugar or sugar-free muesli

Wholegrain cereal, such as bran, with fruit or yoghurt

1 slice wholemeal toast topped with fruit spread or peanut butter

1 slice wholemeal toast or pitta bread, with scrambled or poached eggs

Porridge made with semi-skimmed milk and topped with fresh or dried fruit

Whole-grain bagel with low-fat soft cheese

Replace fried bacon and eggs with grilled turkey rashers and poached eggs

Fluids - Water

Physical thirst can actually fool our bodies into thinking that we're tired – so when we think we need a rest, our bodies may actually be in need of water. It is believed that even slight dehydration can make us feel tired and lethargic. Drinking plenty of water to keep hydrated and energised is a must, the current recommendation being 8 glasses of water a day.

Whilst exercising, it is vital to replace fluid lost through sweating, so ensure that you're not thirsty to start with and don't wait until you're thirsty to have a drink.

Fluids - Alcohol

Consume less alcohol. Alcohol may make us fall asleep initially, but it is actually a stimulant and interferes with natural, restful sleep regardless of how many hours we may sleep for.

Cut down on alcohol consumption, especially during the evening, and your body will feel more rested and energised the next day.

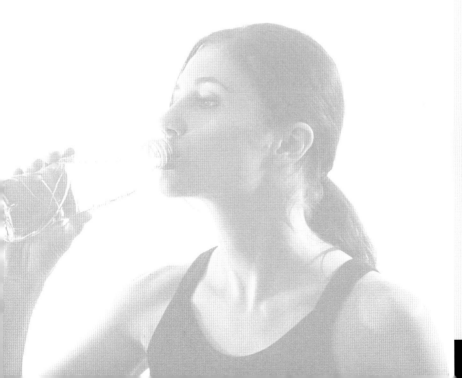

Magnesium

This important mineral has many functions within the body, including breaking down glucose into energy. So if magnesium levels are low within your body you may experience an energy dip. To boost your magnesium level increase your intake of whole grains; especially bran, eat more fish and add a handful of hazelnuts, cashews or almonds to your daily diet.

Snacking the right way

Snacking on fatty or sugary, calorie-empty foods are a surefire way to give your body instant gratification followed quickly by an energy crash, leaving you feeling lethargic and probably in need of another snack. And of course we know all too well the affects on our bodies of having another snack! But if we snack in the right way it can serve to give our metabolism a welcome boost. Foods such as whole grains, nuts and seeds, raw vegetables dipped in humous or salsa, low fat yoghurt, low-fat vegetable soups, (preferably something 'hearty' like lentil soup), or a wholemeal bagel topped with peanut butter or tahini. These types of foods provide a steady release of bodily fuel; so that energy levels are balanced and consistent, avoiding those energy dips that leave us wanting more.

Be organised and buy snacks in small packs, and/or prepare your snacks when you're getting ready for bed the night before. Not only will these foods provide you with important nutrients and energy, but they'll also probably save you money!

Stress

Whether suffered in an acute episode or chronically over time, stress is a huge drain of energy, leaving us potentially exhausted; especially when we don't deal with the underlying cause. Be aware of your reaction to stress and find a suitable way for you to unwind and relax. Relaxation reduces tension and will thus aid energy levels. Look at the previous chapter for methods of relaxtion.

Take a nap

Research has shown that taking a 20 minute power-nap can help increase energy levels, improve memory retention, curb negative emotional responses and reverse the effects of pushing ourselves, both physically and mentally, too hard.

Energise

The effect that our diets can have on how we look, feel and operate is an accepted part of modern thinking. But sometimes the overload of information, faddy diets and well-intentioned advice can be overwhelming and we're left not knowing which eating plan to follow! So, imagine what it might be like to incorporate into your diet a set of 'superfoods' powerful enough to lower cholesterol, aid digestion, protect against a range of diseases and illnesses, alleviate stress and even enhance how we look. A healthy diet incorporating a variety of 'superfoods' is thought to help prevent disease, increase fitness levels and help us to live longer, more energised lives.

Superfoods
Advances in research have uncovered the benefits of certain food types, or 'superfoods' which are believed to be nutrient dense foods.

Containing a broad spectrum of beneficial macro and micro-nutrients that aid the body in generating healthy cells, these foods are thought to help us achieve optimum physical and mental health if eaten regularly, and as part of an overall healthy lifestyle.

The high levels of antioxidants contained in superfoods are a class of vitamins, minerals and enzymes that help the body to fight cell damage from free radicals, believed to play a part in the ageing process, and a contributory factor in chronic ailments such as cancer, heart disease and other degenerative diseases.

Besides tasting fantastic, superfoods are all natural, unprocessed foods readily available from our local produce providers, outdoor and indoor markets and supermarkets. Tried and tested, they've been consumed for years, with no side effects or toxicity.

Please remember that it is always wise to consult your healthcare provider before making any significant changes in your dietary habits.

Top 10 Superfoods

10 fabulous superfoods and their disease-combating, health-improving benefits. Plus delicious recipes to enjoy.

Beans / Legumes

An excellent source of complex carbohydrates, beans are great for many health reasons; weight loss, lowering cholesterol, preventing heart disease, damaged cell repair and eradicating the body of toxins. Adzuki, mung, fava, soy, lentils… there are an abundance of tasty, nutritious beans to be tried and an exciting array of delicious recipes.

Mixed Bean Soup (Serves 6 - 8)

100g/1/2 cup Haricot beans, soaked overnight and drained
100g/1/2 cup Chick peas, soaked overnight and drained
100g/1/2 cup brown or green lentils, washed, drained
3 ltrs water
450g/1 lb tomatoes tinned or quartered
1 medium onion
1/2 teaspoon turmeric
1 teaspoon ground coriander
3 tablespoons flour
juice 1 lemon
salt and pepper to taste

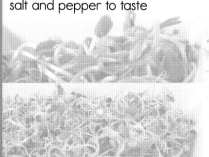
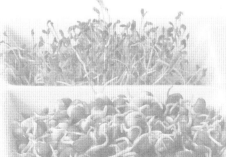

Directions

Put beans, peas and lentils in the water and boil. Reduce heat and simmer for 1 hour or until pulses are tender.

Add tomatoes, onions, turmeric and coriander and leave for 1/2 hour then beat flour and 175ml/3/4 cup water into a smooth paste and stir in. Cook for another 15 minutes or until pulses are soft and just breaking up, add more water if necessary. Adjust the seasoning, stir in lemon juice and serve.

Adzuki Beans and Kale

225ml/1 cup uncooked adzuki beans
1 tablespoon olive oil
2 cloves garlic, peeled and crushed
1.5kg/6 cups roughly chopped kale
2 tablespoons water
55ml/1/4 cup of tamari *
1 teaspoon ground cumin
1 teaspoon ground coriander
salt and pepper to taste

Directions

Place adzuki beans in a pan with enough water to cover. Bring to a boil and then simmer for 30 to 45 minutes, until the beans are tender.

Heat the olive oil over a medium heat, and saute the garlic for about 1 minute. Mix in the kale and 2 tablespoons water.

Season and blend in the tamari, cumin, and coriander with the beans. Reduce the heat to low, cover, and simmer for about another 20 minutes, until the kale is tender. Season with salt and pepper.

* Tamari is a type of soy sauce that is made without wheat. It is dark in colour and has a rich flavour, making it useful in marinades and dressings. It's also good as a dip. If you can't find it, substitute dark soy sauce.

Blueberries

Blueberries are packed with antioxidants, potassium and vitamin C. Ranking high on the list of superfoods, blueberries are high in compounds that help to protect the heart and may even reduce the risk of cancer cells.

They are also an anti-inflammatory, which aids in combating many chronic inflammatory illnesses.

Other benefits include strengthening the immune system, guarding against neurological disorders, improving age-related neurological functioning, protecting eyesight and warding off urinary tract infections.

Super-berry smoothie (serves 2)

115g/1 cup of blueberries
115g/1 cup of raspberries
225ml/1 cup of cranberry juice
60g/1/2 cup of non-fat vanilla yoghurt
1 tbsp unsweetened dark chocolate cocoa powder

Directions
Mix all ingredients in a blender until smooth and pour.

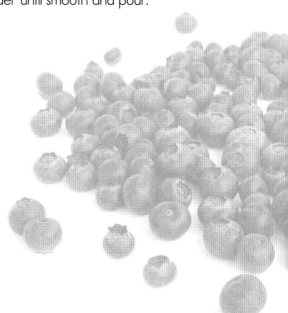

Blueberry Cheesecake With Peaches

200g/1 cup crushed digestive biscuits
75g/3 oz melted butter
250g/2 cups blueberries
110g/1/2 cup granulated sugar
juice of 1 lemon
5 leaves gelatine
400g/1 3/4 cup mascarpone
400g/1 3/4 cup cream cheese
225ml/1 cup cream
50g/1/4 cup icing sugar
4 peaches

Directions

Mix together the digestive biscuits and the melted butter and then press into a springform cake tin. Refrigerate.

Boil the blueberries, granulated sugar and lemon juice until the blueberries are soft. Soak 5 leaves gelatine in cold water for 5 minutes and then add to the hot blueberries.

Whip the cream cheese and mascarpone together with the icing sugar then add the cream and whip. Fold in the blueberry mixture. Then pour into the base. Chill for at least 6 hours, preferably overnight.

Remove the skin from the peaches, then cut them in half, remove stone and slice into segments. Serve on top of the cheesecake.

To make it easier to skin the peaches, score the top of each peach with a sharp knife and then plunge into boiling water. Remove after 5 seconds and plunge into ice cold water.

Caution: Do not put your hands directly in either the boiling or the ice cold water. Fish out the peaches with a ladle.

Broccoli

Broccoli is still one of the most abundant foods containing disease-fighting antioxidants. Broccoli has a spectacular array of health benefits; high anti-cancer activity, cholesterol reducing, anti-viral and anti-ulcer, insulin and blood sugar regulating and an effective anti-inflammatory.

Broccoli with garlic and pine nuts (serves 4-5)

1.5kg/5 cups of broccoli florets
6 cloves of garlic, chopped finely
3 tablespoon olive oil
55g/1/4 cup hazelnuts
Salt - to taste

Directions
Steam the broccoli for 4-5 minutes. Whilst steaming, heat the olive oil over a medium heat and add the pine nuts to toast lightly for about 1-2 minutes.

Add the chopped garlic and continue to heat for another minute. Add the broccoli to the pan and coat with the olive oil mixture, cook for a further 3-4 minutes until softened
to preferred taste.
Add salt to taste
if required.

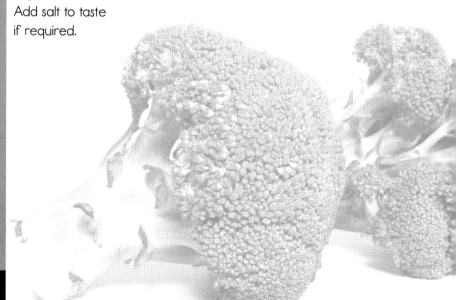

Superfoods

Dolcelatte and Broccoli Quiche (serves 4)

225g/8oz cheese shortcrust pastry
1 teaspoon chopped onions
75g/3oz broccoli florets
75g/3oz Dolcelatte cheese, grated
175g/6oz natural yoghurt
2 eggs
Salt and black pepper

Directions

Preheat the oven to 200C, 400F, Gas mark 6. Roll out the pastry and use to line a 20cm/8 inch flan case. Line with greaseproof paper, fill with baking beans and bake for 15 minutes. Meanwhile, bring a large pan of water to the boil, add the broccoli florets and blanch for 4 minutes. Sprinkle the onions and Dolcelatte over the pastry base, and arrange the broccoli florets on top. Beat together the yogurt and eggs, season to taste and pour into the flan case. Return to the oven and bake for 25-30 minutes, until set and golden.

Cream of Broccoli Soup (serves 4 as a starter)

2 tablespoons butter
1 medium onion, chopped
230g/2 cups broccoli florets
675ml/3 cups vegetable stock
2 tablespoons plain flour
450ml/2 cups milk
salt and white pepper powder to taste

Directions

Heat half the butter in a pan and saute the onions lightly then add the broccoli and stir-fry till glossy. Add the stock and cook for about 4 minutes or till the broccoli is tender. Cool and make a puree. In another pan, heat the remaining butter on low heat till just melted. Add the plain flour and stir well for about only a minute then add the milk and bring to a boil. Simmer for about 5 minutes. Mix in the salt and white pepper powder. Pour in the puree and heat through.

Containing more vitamin C than oranges, more beta-carotene than carrots and providing a good source of B vitamins, antioxidants and amino acids; goji berries are believed to help fight heart disease, boost our immune systems, protect our skin from sun damage and defend our bodies against cancer.

Rum, Goji Berry & Chocolate Ice Cream

100g/1/2 cup Goji Berries soaked in rum for 4 hours
3 Egg yolks
175g/3/4 cup sugar
300ml/1 3/4 cup milk
100g/1/2 cup grated plain chocolate
1 teaspoon vanilla extract
450ml/2 cups whipping cream, softly whipped

Directions

Whisk the egg yolks, sugar, and milk in a bowl over a double boiler (hot water) until smooth – do not boil. Stir in the goji berries and chocolate, then carefully fold in the whipped cream. Transfer the mixture to a plastic container and freeze for one hour, before taking it out and beating the mixture. Freeze for another hour and beat again. Freeze a final time until the mixture is needed. Remove from the freezer approx. 20 minutes prior to serving.

Pumpkin and Goji Fritter

75g/1/3 cup goji berries
450g/1 lb fresh pumpkin
4 tablespoon caster sugar
125g/3/4 cup self raising flour
1 teaspoon orange rind (or a table spoon of mixed peel, finely chopped)
1/2 teaspoon ground allspice
2 eggs (separated)
sunflower oil for deep fat frying
ground cinnamon

Directions
Soak the goji berries in water to rehydrate them and then chop the pumpkin into small cubes and discard the seeds. Boil for 10 minutes or until tender. Drain off water and mash.

Drain the berries and mix with the mashed pumpkin, 2 tablespoons of sugar, flour, orange, egg yolks, and allspice. Beat the egg whites until stiff, then fold into pumpkin mixture.

Heat the oil in a frying pan until very hot then drop in a dollop of the mixture and cook for 8 – 10 minutes so they are golden brown. Drain on some kitchen towel. Dust with cinnamon and sugar. Best served warm.

Goji Jam
50g/1/4 cup Goji berries, soaked, keep and use soak water
1/2 teaspoon orange zest
1/2 teaspoon grated fresh ginger
1 pitted date or 1 teaspoon raw honey

Directions
Combine all of the ingredients together in a blender and mix until pureed. You can also add 1 cup of coconut milk or purified water to create an energy juice drink.

Nuts and seeds are high in essential fatty acids, (good fats) and dense in nutrients essential for our good health including; vitamins A, B, C and E, calcium, zinc, potassium, iron, folic acid, selenium and magnesium.

Eat nuts and seeds such as linseeds, sunflower seeds, alfalfa seeds, pumpkin seeds, almonds, pecans, brazil nuts, cashews and walnuts. You don't need to eat a lot of them, just a small amount in the palm of your hand daily.

Muesli Bars
55g/1/2 cup of unsalted butter
45g/1/4 cup brown sugar
3 tablespoons honey
225ml/1 cup quick cooking oats
55g/1/4 cup of chopped hazelnuts (macadamias, almonds - optional)
55g/1/4 cup of shredded coconut
55g/1/4 cup of sesame seeds

Directions
Preheat the oven to 180 degrees C and grease a baking pan, ready for the mixture.

Combine the butter, brown sugar and honey in a pan, over a low heat until the butter is melted and sugar has dissolved.

Remove from the heat and add the oats, nuts, coconut and sesame seeds. Mix with a wooden spoon until well combined. Press mixture evenly into the prepared baking pan.

Bake for between 15-20 minutes, until the top is golden brown. Let cool in the pan and cut into bars.

Superfoods

Cashew Nut Roast with Sage and onion stuffing

30g/1/6 cup of butter
2 sticks of celery, finely chopped
1 medium leek, finely chopped
330ml/1 1/2 cups of hot water
1 teaspoon of yeast extract (marmite, vegemite etc.)
550g/3 cups of ground cashew nuts
2 tablespoons of soya flour
2 teaspoons of fresh herbs
160g/3 cups of white bread crumbs
sea salt and pepper to taste

Directions

Melt the butter and cook the celery and leek in it for a few minutes. Mix the yeast extract into the hot water and add this to the leek and celery. Stir in the soya flour, nuts, herbs, breadcrumbs and salt and pepper and mix well. Allow to cool slightly while you grease a loaf tin.

Place half the nut roast mixture in the tin and press down well - then add the sage and onion stuffing (pressing down well again) and place the rest of the mixture on top. Bake in the oven for 40 minutes at 180 degrees C.

For the stuffing:
6 slices of wholemeal bread
85g/3oz of butter
4 teaspoons of dried sage or 8 of fresh
1 finely chopped large onion
salt to taste

Melt the butter in a saucepan and then cook the onion in it until soft. Break up the wholemeal bread into fairly small pieces and then mix into the onion and butter with the sage and salt.

Omega-3 fatty acids

Active in protecting our bodies against heart disease and lowering the risk of heart attacks and strokes, omega-3 fats are an essential part of our daily diets.

They also have immune enhancing and anti-inflammatory properties, which are known to reduce the risk of certain cancers and alleviate some of the symptoms of rheumatoid arthritis.

It is also believed that omega-3 fats may help with memory loss and improve cognitive function. Aiming for 2-3 portions per week, fish such as wild salmon, tuna, herring, sardines and trout all contain omega-3 fatty acids.

Grilled Salmon and Avocado Dip (serves 2)
2 salmon steaks
2 avocados - peeled, pitted and diced
2 cloves garlic - peeled and ground
3 tablespoons Greek-style yogurt
1 tablespoon fresh lemon juice
salt and pepper to taste
2 teaspoons dried dill weed
2 teaspoons lemon pepper

Directions
Mash the avocados, garlic, yogurt, and lemon juice together in a bowl. Season lightly with salt and pepper.

Lightly rub the salmon with dill, lemon, pepper and salt. Place under the grill, and cook 15 for minutes, turning once, or until easily flaked with a fork.

Serve with the avocado mixture.

Superfoods

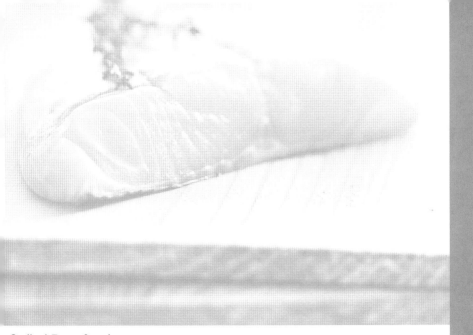

Grilled Tuna Steaks

4 tuna steaks
3 tablespoons of lime juice
2 tablespoons of soy sauce
1 tablespoons of garlic, minced
1 tablespoon of ginger, minced
Lime slices, to serve with

Directions

Place the tuna steaks in a suitably sized casserole dish. In a bowl mix together the lime juice, soy sauce, garlic and ginger then pour evenly over the tuna steaks. Allow to marinate in your refrigerator for at least 2 hours.

Remove the tuna steaks from the marinade and cook under a medium to hot grill for about 8 minutes, turning once. Serve with lime slices. This recipe is complimented by simple couscous or noodles.

If you would like to bar-b-que your tuna steaks, spray the grill with oil to prevent the tuna from sticking and place the rack about 6 inches from the coals. Again, grill for around 8 minutes.

Superfoods

Pomegranate

Pomegranate juice contains the highest antioxidant capacity compared to any other juice. These powerful free radical fighting properties support good cholesterol levels and healthy coronary artery function. Pomegranates have been found to actively reduce the risk of cardio-vascular disease.

Spiced Pears and Pomegranate (serves 2-3)
1 pomegranate, skin and light-coloured membrane removed
3 pears - peeled, cored and cut into wedges
1 tablespoon fresh lemon juice
2 tablespoon light brown sugar
1/4 teaspoon ground nutmeg
1/2 teaspoon ground cinnamon
2 tablespoon finely chopped almonds
4 sprigs fresh mint leaves for garnish

Directions

Put the pomegranate seeds and pear slices into a bowl and toss them with lemon juice until thoroughly coated.

Mix the nutmeg, brown sugar and cinnamon in a small bowl, then mix into the fruit bowl.

Cover the mixture and refrigerate for at least 1 hour before serving.

Serve in individual dishes, and decorate with a sprinkling of chopped almonds and a sprig of mint, if desired.

Superfoods

Quinoa

Quinoa is a South American grain containing all 9 essential amino acids, constituting it as a complete protein. Far easier to digest than meat, quinoa also has a lower fat content.

An excellent source of fibre, essential fatty acids and abundant in vitamins and minerals, quinoa is fast becoming a popular and more readily available health food.

Quinoa on sale in the UK is yellow, but it is also possible to get red quinoa. Overall a tasty and versatile food that can be used in both savoury and sweet dishes.

Quinoa fruit salad
225ml/1 cup of quinoa – rinsed and drained
225ml/1 cup of water
225ml/1 cup of apple juice
2 red apples, diced
1/2 teaspoon cinnamon
225ml/1 cup of chopped celery
115ml/1/2 cup of dried cranberries
115ml1/2 cup of chopped walnuts
225ml/1 cup of non-fat vanilla yoghurt

Directions
Place the quinoa, apple juice, water and cinnamon in a pan and bring to the boil. Reduce the heat and simmer until all of the liquid is absorbed, (this should take approx 10-15 mins).

Allow the mixture to cool and transfer to a large mixing bowl. Cover the bowl and refrigerate for at least 1 hour.

When ready, add the apples, celery, dried cranberries and walnuts and mix well. Carefully fold in the yoghurt and serve immediately.

Superfoods

Quinoa Risotto (serves 6)
225ml/1 cup quinoa
1 tablespoon olive oil
225ml/1 cup chopped onion
3 cloves garlic, minced
225ml/1 cup vegetable broth
225ml/1 cup skim milk
225g/8 oz. mushrooms, sliced
165ml/3/4 cup Parmesan cheese
Rinse and drain quinoa three times, using a fine mesh strainer to remove the bitter outer coating.

Directions
Heat olive oil in a heavy saucepan or dutch oven over medium-high heat. Add onion and cook until soft, stirring constantly. Add garlic and quinoa and continue stirring a minute or two. Stir in broth and milk. Bring to a boil, then reduce heat to low and simmer until quinoa is tender, stirring occasionally, approximately 10-12 minutes.

Add mushrooms and cook another 3-5 minutes, stirring often. Remove from heat. Add cheese and let stand a few minutes, so risotto can thicken.

Believed to help lower cholesterol and lower the risk of heart disease, soy is a popular choice for a healthy lifestyle. Good sources of soy are found in tofu, soy milk.

Breaded, Fried, Softly Spiced Tofu
1 pack of extra-firm tofu, drained and pressed
450ml/2 cups of vegetable stock
3 tablespoons vegetable oil
1/2 teaspoon cayenne pepper
75g/1/2 cup of plain flour
3 tablespoon yeast
1 teaspoon salt
1/2 teaspoon freshly ground black pepper
1 teaspoon sage

Directions
Cut the tofu into 1/2 inch thick slices; then cut again into 1/2 inch wide sticks. Place the tofu in a bowl, pour the vegetable stock over the top and set aside to soak.

To make the breading mixture, stir together the flour, yeast, salt, pepper, sage, and cayenne. Warm the vegetable oil over a medium heat.

Remove the tofu sticks from the stock, and squeeze out most (but not all) of the liquid from them. Roll the sticks in the breading mixture, making sure you have good coverage of the mixture.

Place the tofu in the heated oil; fry the tofu until crisp and browned on all sides. Serve with a mixed salad.

Superfoods

Tomatoes are loaded with lycopene, which gives the tomato its rich red colour. Lycopene is an antioxidant which has been found to boost the immune system, be heart-healthy and reduce the risk of prostate, breast, lung and other cancers. The absorption of lycopene is optimum when tomatoes are cooked in olive oil.

Pesto Tomatoes
10 small ripe tomatoes
115ml/1/2 cup homemade or purchased pesto
225ml/1 cup grated Parmesan cheese

Directions
Preheat the oven to 180 degrees C. Slice the tomatoes in half and scoop out about a tablespoon of flesh from the centre of each half. Fill the scooped out pocket with pesto, and sprinkle generously with the parmesan cheese. Place the tomato halves in a well oiled (olive oil) baking dish and bake in the oven until the cheese is melted and slightly browned.

Tomato, basil and couscous salad (serves 6)
500ml/2 1/4 cups chicken stock
275g/10 oz box couscous
225ml/1 cup chopped spring onions
225ml/1 cup diced seeded plum tomatoes
75ml/1/3 cup thinly sliced fresh basil
75ml/1/2 cup olive oil
55ml/1/4 cup balsamic vinegar
55ml/1/4 teaspoon dried crushed red pepper
cherry tomatoes, halved
basil leaves for garnish

Directions
Bring the stock to boil in medium saucepan and add the couscous. Remove from the heat, cover and let stand 5 minutes. Transfer to a large bowl, fluff with a fork and allow to cool. Mix all of the ingredients except the cherry tomatoes into the couscous. Season with salt and pepper. Garnish with cherry tomatoes and basil leaves.

Superfoods

Tomato, olive oil and fresh bean sauce (serves 4)
800g/2 lbs (approx) fresh green beans, trimmed
150ml/3/4 cup extra virgin olive oil
1 large onion, cut into thin slices
2 garlic cloves, finely chopped
2 small potatoes, peeled and cut into small cubes
675g fresh tomatoes or 400 g canned tomatoes, finely chopped
150ml/2/3 of a cup hot water
3-4 tablespoon finely chopped fresh parsley
salt & pepper to taste

Directions
Cut the fresh beans in half, if too long and place in a bowl filled with cold water. Sautee the onion in plenty of olive oil, add the garlic and as soon as it begins to give off a smell, throw in the cubed potatoes. After a couple of minutes have passed, add the tomatoes and hot water and allow it to boil for 5 minutes.

Next, wash the fresh beans well and add them to the boiling content of your stewpot, seasoning with salt and pepper according to taste. Cover the pot and simmer for about 30 minutes. Sprinkle with finely chopped parsley and if needed, add extra hot water. Cook another 10 minutes, until the beans are very tender. Serve hot with a big piece of feta cheese.

Tomato Salad

6 fresh ripe tomatoes
6 sprigs of fresh finely chopped oregano (or dried)
sea salt
black ground pepper (optional)
extra virgin olive oil

Directions

Wash and dry the tomatoes then slice in 1/4 to 1/2 inch slices and arrange on serving dish. Sprinkle the tomatoes with the oregano, sea salt, and freshly ground pepper to taste.

Drizzle with your best quality olive oil and serve at room temperature.

Tomato Bruschetta (serves 2 as a starter)

4 slices Italian or French country-style bread – in thick slices
extra virgin olive oil
5 medium-sized ripe juicy tomatoes
sea salt

Directions

Cut 4 thick slices of bread and toast both sides of the slices in a toaster, or under a grill. Place the toast on a large plate without stacking them.

Cut a tomato in half crosswise and rub the cut side of the tomato onto each toast. First you do one side, turn the toast over, and rub the tomato on the other side of the toast. Use one tomato per piece of toast and make sure that you rub all toast with the tomato halves.

Drizzle olive oil liberally onto both sides of the toast. Finally, sprinkle some salt over the slices of bread to taste.

Finely chop the remaining tomato and use as garnish for the bruschetta.

Our skin is the world's window into our personal health, vitality and emotional wellbeing. Radiant and glowing skin shows good health, vitality and personal care. Dull and tired looking skin shows an unhealthy lifestyle, stress and a lack of overall care. Natural beauty and skin is available for us all – it doesn't have to be in a salon, over a make-up counter, with a plastic surgeon or in a day spa – but in simple, affordable, remedies and ideas that anyone can follow.

Skin – reflecting what's on the inside

We can apply the most expensive topical skin lotions and potions to our skin, but still not have the vibrant, healthy skin that we want.

This is because the most important factor in how we look on the outside is what we process through our bodies on the inside. This naturally refers to the food and drink that we consume, but also to other environmental factors such as the chemicals that we breathe into our systems – car emissions, carbon monoxide, detergents, cleaning products, fragrances etc.

Some of these factors are beyond our control, but we can certainly prevent unnecessary damage and strive to improve our physiological wellbeing in order to obtain young, healthy, radiant looking skin – literally treating our bodies from the "inside-out"

Skin-friendly food

By far the best start is to take a good look at what we eat. Your finest skin care range is right there in your fridge and food cupboards! Research shows that a nutritionally rich diet slows down the physiological ageing processes in all our tissues, including the skin.

A balanced diet for fabulous skin should include all the nutrients needed to promote good health; protein, carbohydrates, fats, essential fatty acids and all the essential vitamins and minerals. Fresh foods are of optimum importance for your skin, the fresher the better.

Eat liberal amounts of fresh fruit and vegetables, which contain a wide variety of antioxidants; particularly important for the prevention of premature skin ageing. Seeds, nuts and whole grains, accompanied by protective foods like vegetable oils, yogurt, honey and yeast are all skin-friendly foods.

Chicken, fish, eggs, turkey and soy are all good sources of protein and B vitamins. Our modern diets are often lacking in essential B vitamins which are pivotal to healthy hair, nails and skin.

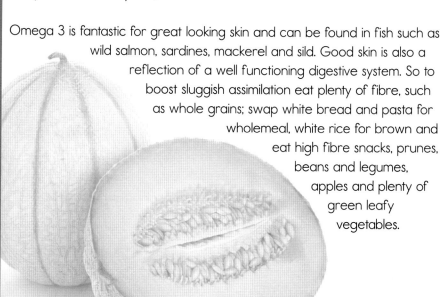

Omega 3 is fantastic for great looking skin and can be found in fish such as wild salmon, sardines, mackerel and sild. Good skin is also a reflection of a well functioning digestive system. So to boost sluggish assimilation eat plenty of fibre, such as whole grains; swap white bread and pasta for wholemeal, white rice for brown and eat high fibre snacks, prunes, beans and legumes, apples and plenty of green leafy vegetables.

A well as eating the right foods, reduce types of food that can deprive the skin of moisture, such as alcohol and caffeine. Avoid processed food whenever possible as they often contain empty-calories, are high in salt and sugar content and lack the valuable nutrients that our bodies crave. Excess sugar is considered to cause premature ageing, damaging protein molecules in the skin and leading to a loss of skin elasticity, causing wrinkles and sagging.

If we invest in a nutritionally balanced diet, we will not only look better but also feel healthy and invigorated. When we feel healthy, we feel good about ourselves and this translates to how we interact with people around us. Try it, see if your nearest and dearest notice the difference!

Essential skincare tips

Blackheads
To loosen blackheads for easier removal, mix equal parts of baking soda and water in your hand and rub gently onto skin for 2 to 3 minutes. Rinse off with warm water.

Boost your circulation
Energise your skin, as well as your body and mind and get yourself moving! Sluggish circulation can affect how your skin looks, worsening bloating and puffiness, cellulite, acne, loss of muscle tone and paleness. Exercise opens up blood vessels to make skin look healthy and youthful. Taking regular cardiovascular exercise increases blood flow to the skin which in turn assists the production of collagen.

So become more active, walk, jog, workout, go to the gym, take a class, even do stretches at work. As well as promoting good circulation physical exertion also helps us to de-stress, which is good for our overall health.

Cosmetics
Regularly replace your cosmetics and cosmetic brushes and sponges, including the sponge in your compact. Generally cosmestics don't have a shelf life of much longer than 6 months to a year, so no matter how tempted you are to hold on to that favourite mascara renew your make-up regularly.

Drink lots of water

Water hydrates our bodies and purifies our insides, aiding the elimination process which will show through in how our skin looks. So remember your 8 glasses per day! Although, take care not drink too much fluid 2-3 hours before going to bed as this may contribute to morning puffiness.

Dry skin brushing

Dry skin brushing is another useful way to boost circulation and to stimulate the lymphatic system. Dry skin brushing exfoliates the skin, getting rid of dead skin cells and allowing the skin to detox more effectively. It also tightens skin, promotes removal of cellulite and increases skin renewal and rejuvenation. Best carried out just before taking a shower in the morning, you'll need a natural bristle brush, (not synthetic) preferably with a long handle in order to reach all parts of the body. Don't wet the skin beforehand as this stretches the skin. Start at the soles of the feet and work up your legs, to your abdomen, buttocks, back and lastly hands to arms. Brush the skin from each part of your body towards the heart.

When brushing the abdomen make circular anti-clockwise strokes, be gentle around the breast area and avoid the nipples. Brush each body part several times before showering or bathing in warm water.

Rinse at the end with a cool rinse to invigorate circulation.

Dryness
Scratch a small area of skin on your arm with a fingernail, if it leaves a white mark then your skin is dry and needs exfoliating and moisturising.

Hands and feet
For luxuriously soft skin, use an intensive moisturising cream on your hands and feet at night and then wear thin-fabric gloves and socks. Keep them on overnight to achieve best results.

Ingredients
Skin products with ingredients containing fragrances, dyes and preservatives can be too harsh for certain skin types. Sensitive skin is particularly easily damaged and takes longer to recover.

Be wary of alcohol-based products, as these can disturb the pH level of our complexions, leaving it dry and dehydrated.

Lose the flannel
Traditional washcloths and flannels are too abrasive to use on the face, so use your hands and fingers instead.

Mixing different skincare products
It's easy to collect an array of different skincare products, but probably not the most effective way to care for your skin. You may be using products that contain the same ingredients, so are either on overkill or paying for something that you already have.

The other consideration is that some of the products may be incompatible and react unfavourably together. It's better to stick with a good brand name and use their range of products.

Moist, hot skin
To keep areas of the body that are prone to getting hot and sweaty, clean and dry, use un-perfumed baby powder. Areas such as underarms, inner thighs, bottom cheeks, under the breast area. This will prevent the growth of bacteria or fungi which can cause unpleasant skin conditions.

Natural born skin-killers!

To be avoided at all costs! Smoking, tanning salons, and sunbathing. Each of these horrors age the skin prematurely and lead to deep set facial lines - especially draw lines around the mouth area for smokers.

Olive oil

Massage a few drops over your face, backs of your arms, knees and elbows in the evening. This will moisten your skin beautifully.

Out in the sun

If you're out for a day in the sun, don't wear scented lotions and perfumes. This can lead to blotchy and itchy skin. Neither attractive, or comfortable!

Seasonal changes

During the winter our skin needs more moisture than summer, so reflect this in the products you use, i.e. a lighter moisturiser in summer and a heavier one for winter.

Sleep

Essential to our overall health, it is also vital to our skin because the majority of cell repair and regeneration occurs whilst we are sleeping. So if we're not getting enough kip our skin can't work effectively at repairing itself.

Steaming

Steam opens the skin's pores while deeply cleansing and rejuvenating all the skin's layers. Using herbs in facial steams is a great way to nourish your skin. Therapeutic herbs can be added to the water so that their healing benefits will become part of the steam and reach deep into your pores. Many herbs are emollient, softening and lubricating; others hydrate and moisturize; most are antibacterial and anti-inflammatory.

Licorice root is the number one herbal choice for steaming as it suits all skin types, by opening the pores, soothing, cleansing, and lubricating. As for other herbs, for dry skin try lavender or mint; for sensitve skin try chamomile and for oily skin try mint, lavender, rose and/or witch hazel.
Here are simple, seven-step directions to make your own facial steam:

Stop touching!

Our hands are usually our primary form of bodily contact, consequently they are a breeding ground for dirt and germs.

When we touch our faces we're transferring the contents of our hands to our face! Not a pleasant thought, or at all good for our complexions.

Turn down the heat

Hot showers and baths strip skin of its moisture and wash away protective oils, so avoid using hot water and use lukewarm instead, to prevent over-drying of the skin.

Vitamins

Products containing vitamins are becoming increasingly more popular. Vitamin A, for fine lines and wrinkles, vitamin B for glowing skin and moisture retention, vitamin C for repairing sun damage and enhancing collagen production, vitamin E for powerful moisturising properties and repairing dry, rough skin and vitamin K for reducing dark circles under the eyes.

Wash your face

It is important to wash your face in the morning and at night. When we sleep yucky stuff like dead skin cells, dirt, and dust accumulates so wash off the overnight nasties first thing in the morning!

Completely natural skin remedies

Simple, homemade skin therapies for achieving luminous, beautiful skin. And you'll smell good too!

Apple Tonic (for all skin types)
Take a quarter cup of organic apple juice and apply to the face with a cotton ball. Leave for a few minutes then rinse.

Apples contain a natural fruit acid which has an exfoliating effect. For oily skin add half a teaspoon of lime to the apple juice.

Avocado Moisturiser (for dry skin)
Take the skin of an avocado and smooth it all over your face, avoiding the eyes and nose. Allow to set for 15 minutes before rinsing off.

Banana and honey cream (for all skin types)
Mash 1/2 a banana, mix in 1 tablespoon honey and 2 tablespoons of sour cream. Apply to the face and allow to set for about 10 minutes, then gently rinse off.

Brown Sugar Body Exfoliant
Mix half a cup of brown sugar, 1 tablespoon of vitamin E oil and half a freshly squeezed orange in a bowl.

Stand in the bath or shower and wet your body. Taking handfuls of the mixture gently scrub over your body in circular motions. When all areas of the body have been scrubbed, rinse off and dry as normal. Apply a moisturising lotion once dried to prevent your skin dehydrating.

Cucumber Refresher (for all skin types)
Grate or blend a cucumber and apply over the face and around the eyes. Leave for 15 to 20 minutes and rinse off.

Lime Juice Eye-Reviver
Take 4 tablespoons of lime juice and iced water. Saturate cotton pads in the mixture and place over closed eyelids for 10 minutes.

Milk & Honey Oatmeal Cleanser (for all skin types)
Mix ½ cup ground oatmeal, ½ cup milk and 1 tablespoon of honey.

Once mixed, massage into the skin gently, then rinse off with lukewarm water. Refrigerate any remaining mixture after use.

Orange and Yogurt Vibrancy Mask (for combination skin)
Mix the grated rind of one orange with ½ cup of organic yogurt.

Apply to the face and wait 10 minutes before rinsing off.

Strawberry Purifier (for oily skin)
Mix ¼ cup pure aloe vera, 2 tablespoons of plain organic yoghurt, three crushed strawberries and ¼ cup Borax.

Once mixed, massage gently into skin then rinse off with lukewarm water.

Summer skin care

Summer is one of the seasonal battles for maintaining good skin care! Summer may not have the harsh cold or winds of the winter, but it does have the punishing heat of the sun at its maximum strength during the summer months. To reduce or avoid the effects of the sun's harmful rays, here are a few tips.

Using sunscreen product which has an SPF of 15 or above is essential for us all. Allowing yourself to bake in the midday sun, damages and prematurely ages skin – as well as increasing the risk of skin cancer. Use a complete sun-block of factor 50 for children. Research indicates that one or more severe sunburns in childhood or adolescence can significantly increase the risk of developing skin cancer later in life.

Check the expiry date on your sunscreen. Sunscreen without an expiry date should not be kept for any longer than 3 years.

Always wear a hat in the sun, preferably with a wide brim which will protect your face.

Always wear sunglasses which block 100% of the sun's UV rays. Most retail outlets sell sunglasses with a sticker showing the percentage of UV protection. These will protect your eyes and also the skin around them which is particularly thin.

If you are wearing lightweight or lightly coloured fabrics use sunscreen under your clothing. Research has proven that the sun can penetrate lightweight and lighter coloured fabrics. And if you're not worried about being too hot, wear darker, tightly woven fabrics as these are much more effective at blocking UV rays.

Drink plenty of water, hot weather increases the risk of dehydration which can be very dangerous if an extreme case. If you are undertaking any form of exercise or other physical activity, have a drink before you start and keep drinking throughout. In addition to the health risks of dehydration your skin will take a hammering if your body is lacking essential water.

Skincare

Check your skin

The incidence of skin cancer is on the increase and it is believed that many deaths that occur can be prevented via early detection.

By taking the time to examine your skin monthly, you will become familiar with what is normal for you and where any blemishes and moles are located. It is useful to note down the dates of self-exams.

Check the entirety of your body, including the feet, between the toes and the whole of your head; including your ears and scalp. Use a mirror for parts of your body that are hard to see and make sure that the room has good visibility or is well-lit. Whilst you are looking at each area, use your hands to feel over your skin.

If you are concerned about anything that you find, regardless of how small and how 'silly' you might feel, be sure to make an appointment with your Doctor and get yourself checked out.

For more advice on what to look for you can visit the website www.cancerresearchuk.org.

Skincare

Winter skin care

The cold climate brings with it a range of skin-nightmares - dry, rough, sore, flaky and itchy – not to mention chapped lips! Winter really is your skin's arch-enemy. Follow these tips to reduce the effects of winter on your skin.

Outside the temperature falls and inside the heating goes up! Central heating wreaks havoc on skin, eyes and nasal passages, drying them out and causing discomfort. Have the thermostat set to the lowest level that you can comfortably stand. If you have access to room humidifiers, these will help to balance out the moisture levels in the room. Drink lots of water. Internal hydration keeps skin cells plump and healthy.

Although most of us relish the thought of a hot bath or shower when it's cold, this will dry skin out more. Keep showers and baths short and use warm water, not hot. Use gentle skin products for your skin care, anything too harsh will worsen any already dry and sensitive skin.

Moisturising effectively is essential in winter, so a suitable moisturiser for your skin type is a must. Your winter moisturiser should be heavier than the one that you use for summer as your skin will crave more moisture in the cold. Pay attention to dry areas, hands, feet, elbows and knees so that they don't become cracked and painful.

You will still need protection from the sun in winter, even though it has lost its heat. Remember to protect your ears and lips also.

Exfoliate on a weekly basis with a gentle exfoliating product. This will remove dead skin cells and prevent your skin from looking grey and dull.

Have you ever wondered how some people seem to achieve shiny, healthy, luscious looking hair, sporting an immaculate style which never looks out of place? Ever wondered why you can't achieve the same look? Well, healthy hair is not hard to achieve, or a best-kept secret that no-one has let you in on – all you need to do is learn a few natural, creative and clever hair care tips and you'll be the envy of your friends.

Natural hair care solutions

Avocado
Known for its beneficial proteins and hydrating properties, mash one avocado and mix it with 1 tablespoon of lemon juice, 1 teaspoon of sea salt and 1 tablespoon of pure aloe vera. Mix the ingredients until they turn into a paste and then comb through your hair with your fingers. Cover with a plastic shower cap, (or bag), and wrap a towel around your head. Leave for 20-30 minutes before rinsing out the paste and shampooing as normal.

Baking soda
Need to remove grease, dirt and the gunk of products from your hair without adding even more gunk to it? Add 1 tablespoon of baking soda to your hair while shampooing and it will remove all those nasty chemicals that styling products deposit.

Beer
For a boost of life for your hair use some flat beer. Mix 3 tablespoons of beer in a half cup of warm water and after shampooing and rinsing your hair, rub in the mix gently and leave for a couple of minutes before rinsing it off.

Butter
As a remedy to dry, damaged hair use butter for a glorious shine! Take a small knob of butter and massage it into your dry hair. Cover your hair over with a shower cap for half an hour and then shampoo and rinse as normal.

Castor Oil

For maximum shine for dull hair, mix up 2 teaspoons of castor oil, 1 teaspoon glycerine and one egg white. Massage the mixture into wet hair and wash out after a few minutes.

Espresso

For extra shine make one cup of strong espresso and let it cool. Pour the liquid over your dry hair and leave for 20 minutes. Rinse out as normal.

Lemon juice

Lemon juice mixed with water can be used as a last rinse to give your hair added shine and bounce.

Mayonnaise

For an effective way to condition your hair and give it a naturally gorgeous shine, use a dollop of mayonnaise and massage it into your hair and scalp. Cover your head with a shower cap and wait a few minutes before shampooing out.

Olive Oil

A sleek and fashionable method of putting back much needed moisture and lustre into dry, brittle hair. Apply half a cup of warm, (not hot!), olive oil to your hair, making sure that you massage it well into your hair and scalp. Cover your hair with a cap and leave for 45 minutes before shampooing and rinsing as normal.

Tea

For an old fashioned hair remedy said to add a natural shine to hair, use a litre of warm tea, (without the sugar or milk!), as your final rinse after shampooing.

Vinegar

To make a great conditioner that will inject life into limp or lifeless hair, mix 1 teaspoon of apple cider vinegar, 3 egg whites and 2 tablespoons of olive oil. Massage the mixture into your hair, cover with a cap and leave for 30 minutes before shampooing and rinsing.

Fabulous-Looking Hair Tips

Afro hair or extra curly hair
Avoid using brushes on these types of hair as this can cause damage by pulling out hair from the scalp or breaking the hair part way down. Instead, use a wide toothed comb or even your fingers to work through your hair.

Drink water
Drinking plenty of water will hydrate your skin, body and hair. Dehydration will show on your scalp and in the condition of your hair, so do your best to drink the recommend 8 glasses per day.

Healthy diet
The well-coined phrase "You are what you eat" extends to the condition and health of your hair. For shiny, glowing hair a well balanced diet with plenty of proteins and vitamins will keep your hair and scalp in optimum condition, from the inside out. Vitamins such as biotin, vitamin E, vitamin B and vitamin C are believed to boost hair growth and condition.

Heat protection
Our hair beauty regimes consist of hairdryers, straighteners, curlers, heated rollers and all manner of heat-based methods of styling. Naturally, this dries hair out, stripping it of moisture and leaving hair frazzled, hard to style and worst of all, breaking off. Before using a hairdryer, pat your hair dry with a towel and let the remaining moisture in your hair dry naturally, leaving your hair damp and reducing the amount of blow-drying time.

To further minimise the damage caused by heat styling use a good heat protection product. These can be sourced in good hair salons and it might be useful to ask for advice in purchasing the right product for your hair.

Massage

Massaging your scalp increases the blood flow, nourishing the roots and stimulating hair growth. Some hair and beauty salons offer head massages as part of their treatments. An excellent opportunity to relax, as well as good for your scalp and hair!

Moisturise

For any essential moisturising treatment use either a conditioner especially for intense conditioning at least once a week, or alternatively one of the moisturising natural remedies detailed in this section.

Apply to your hair as normal, but leave on and cover with a shower cap for between 10-20 minutes, (or the recommended treatment time). This will ensure that your hair absorbs valuable moisture, leaving your hair well conditioned and soft to touch.

Product build-up

Too much product in your hair will make it look heavy, tired and dirty. Use a natural method of cleansing product build-up for a fresh start and don't overdo it with products going forward. Generally one product to style and one to give it a last minute finish should be plenty.

Avoid applying hair styling products directly onto your scalp, as this will clog the pores on your head.

Sleep

During our sleep our bodies are catching up on necessary rest and processes of rejuvenation and repair are hard at work, internally and externally. This includes our hair and any damage that has taken place. So sleep is a healthy-hair essential.

Use a satin pillowcase to cut down on hair rubbing and fly-away hair! Avoid sleeping in hair accessories such as scrunchies, etc. as these can lead to hair damage. Elastic bands are an absolute NO at any time of day!

Products to suit

Greasy, dry, frizzy, combination, coloured, permed, heat damaged, blonde, brunette, redhead... there are so many products to choose from. Where do you start?

General rule of thumb is that if your hair is easy to manage, looks shiny, feels healthy and most importantly, you are happy with it – then you must be doing something right and it's likely that the products that you are using suit your hair type. If this isn't the case then it's possible that you need to change your hair products. Visit your preferred salon and get expert advice from a trusted stylist on what will work most effectively for your hair.

Avoid using hair styling products containing alcohol, which dries out hair.

Natural ingredients
If you prefer your hair-care to include natural ingredients look out for products which contain essential oils, vegetable oils and herbs. Essential oils such as lavender and tea tree have naturally antiseptic properties in them and help in the treatment of dandruff. Rosemary and ylang-ylang are believed to aid hair growth. Vegetable oils such as safflower, soybean and olive oil are fantastic for moisturising and conditioning hair.

Professional cuts
For an instantly healthier look for your hair a good professional haircut is a must-have. Split-ends will be removed, your style will be revitalised; or even changed completely!

Getting help and advice on the right texture, colour, style and hair length for you is important, and as your crowning glory you owe it to yourself to give your hair the best treatment possible.

Regular trims and follow up consultations with your stylist will make your hair look as fabulous as you'll feel. Go on – indulge yourself!

Split ends

Split ends, or 'Trichoptlosis' as it is professionally known– the bane of many a woman's life! This is a widespread condition affecting the ends of hair fibres where the protective cuticle has been stripped away, causing ends to split into 2 to 3 parts. The most effective treatment is to cut off the split end fibre.

Typically most people think this is an issue primarily for long hair, but people with short hair can be just as prone if their hair is in bad condition. Causes include not trimming the hair often enough, over-exposure to the sun and heat-damage generated by heat styling products, colouring and waving causing drying out of the hair shaft, chlorine in swimming baths, overly vigorous brushing or back-combing, poor quality brushes/combs and a lack of natural oils reaching the end of the hair shaft; particularly in long hair. The worst thing we can do with split ends is to ignore them. Every time you brush your hair the ends will split more, eventually breaking off and making your hair shorter and shorter, and in dreadful condition.

Useful tips for split ends
First and foremost – ensure that you book in for a trim regularly. A nightmare for anyone growing their hair, but even the tiniest trim will help your hair look healthier and thicker whilst it's growing. And it will avoid the angst of having to lose a few inches of badly split hair once you're 6-months down the line!

Ask your stylist to recommend specialist products which can temporarily seal the splits and catch any potential splits before they occur. Regimentally deep condition your hair at least once a week. Avoid using heat styling where possible and don't over brush or comb your hair. Invest in quality brushes and combs. Be gentle with your hair!

Shampoo and condition your hair after a workout or strenuous exercise. The salt contained in perspiration erodes the hair shaft, causing brittle hair and split ends.

Buy a good protective conditioner, which is specially designed for swimming in chlorine.

Dandruff

Dandruff is quite simply the shedding of dead skin from your scalp at a faster rate than normal, causing white flakes and itching of the scalp. Everyone experiences having a degree of dandruff at one time or another.

The causes of dandruff vary and can include hormone imbalance, poor nutrition or health, improper rinsing-out of shampoo, lack of sleep, stress, exhaustion, poor hygiene, overuse of styling products, excessive cold or heat, allergic reactions.

Although there is no 'cure' for dandruff, there are ways in which you can control and limit its re-occurrence.

Useful tips for eliminating dandruff

The most important consideration in the treatment of this dandruff is to keep the hair and scalp clean so as to reduce the accumulation of dead cells on the scalp.

For mild dandruff, shampooing your hair with a mild shampoo daily should help. Be sure to wash your hair thoroughly, but gently, and ensure all of the shampoo is washed out. Don't use strong shampoos as this can dry out your hair and irritate your scalp, making the dandruff worse.

If this doesn't help, try an anti-dandruff shampoo. Lather and rinse your hair twice, the first wash will clean your scalp, the second will medicate it.

You should see an improvement within a couple of weeks. Your local pharmacy should be able to advise you on which products to use.

For a more natural approach, a teaspoon of fresh lime juice used in the last rinse is believed to be an effective remedy. Not only leaving the hair shiny and glowing, but removing any sticky products and preventing dandruff.

Choosing the right hairstyle for your face

There are literally thousands of ways in
which we can style our hair, but due to our
own unique set of facial features and
shapes we know that not all of us can
wear long flowing tresses, or that short
elf-like-hair-do that looks so feminine on
the girl on the magazine cover, but
makes us look positively boyish in reality!

So, how can we make the most of our
features and our face shapes? None
of our faces are equal – thin, rounded,
angular, soft, long, square. We need to
accentuate the positive and draw
away from facial features we don't like.

Angular Features
To draw away from a sharp or angular
face shape, or features, create a curly or
wavy hairstyle to soften.

Heart shape face
*Face is wide at the temples and hairline, narrowing
to a small delicate chin.*

Try chin-length or longer hairstyles and side partings.
Layers that are swept forward around the upper part
of the face, with a wispy fringe will achieve a more
balanced look by giving your face fullness where it
needs it. A chin-length bob is fabulous for this face shape.

High forehead
A full fringe lying horizontally across the forehead will
cover the forehead area.

Low forehead

Soft fullness at the crown area and strategically placed vertical lines can help to lengthen the face.

Large Nose

Wearing a full hairstyle, whether layered or curls, or an upswept crown make a larger nose less prominent.

Narrow chin

Wearing long hair with fullness or curls at the chin will make the chin seem wider.

Oval face

Slightly narrower at the jawline than at the temples, with a gently rounded hairline.

Luckily, this face shape can wear almost any hairstyle! The even proportion of an oval face gives a balanced look which suits long, short or medium length hairstyles. Just avoid heavy fringes and styles that are brushed onto the face.

Round face

Full-looking face with a round chin and hairline. Widest point is at the cheeks and ears.

Introducing a side parting in the hair will slim and lengthen the face. A hairstyle with fullness and height at the crown, whilst keeping the rest of your hair relatively close to your head, will make your face seem longer and narrower.

Square face or full chin

A strong, square jawline and usually an equally square hairline.

A short hairstyle with fullness or soft curls at the crown area will detract attention from the chin area.

To soften the square appearance of the face, wear layers and wispy looks.

If your hair is straight maybe invest in a body wave, as waves and curls will create an attractive balance to the straight features of your face shape.

Thin face

Long and slender, about the same width at forehead and just below cheekbones. Narrow chin or forehead.

In need of widening, wearing curls or fullness at the sides will create a wider look. Avoid long hair, which will make the face look longer and thinner.

Winter hair tips

Use a conditioner on your hair every day. Deep condition your hair at least once a week. Once your hair is well conditioned and moist, lock in the moisture by running your hair through cold water, this will also give your hair a healthy glow.

Hot oil treatments are very effective conditioners that can help re-hydrate your hair from central heating systems and cold, windy weather.

Try a natural hot oil solution like jojoba. Your stylist may be able to advise you on reliable and effective treatments.

Wear a hat, scarf or cap when outside, in order to protect your hair from the cold and wind. Make sure that whatever you choose to wear isn't too tight as this will adversely affect the circulation in your scalp. Not only a good way of protecting your hair, but a fantastic opportunity to make a fashion statement!

Don't go out with wet or damp hair, not only is this not particularly good for your general health, but if it's cold enough your hair could freeze and literally break off. This applies to the excess water in your hair causing breakage, but also styling products on damp hair.

Reduce the amount of heat generating styling methods, such as blow drying and using straighteners. If you do use them, use a leave in conditioner and/or a good heat protection product.

Don't use very hot water when washing your hair, this is another way that your hair can get dried out and damaged. Use warm or cool water instead.

Protect long hair by wearing it up. Create clean-swept up-does during the winter months to protect your hair from excessive damage.

Summer hair

As much as most of us love to be in the summer sunshine, the sun can cause mayhem with our hair, leaving it dry, brittle and stripped of natural oils. Not to mention the affects of swimming, saltwater and chlorine!

To limit this damage, these tips should allow you to enjoy the sunshine without costing you the health and beauty of your hair.

Summer hair care tips

When out in the sun, wear a cap, headscarf or hat to protect your scalp and hair from the sun.

If you don't want to wear anything on your head, massage in a leave-in conditioner which has an added sunscreen in its ingredients. Don't assume that all hair care products contain SPF agents, so check the label.

If you've come out and have forgotten to protect your hair, you can always put everyday sunscreen in your hair; this will still protect your hair in the same way as it protects your skin. Make sure that you wash it out and rinse well when you get home though.

Before you jump into the pool or wade into the sea for a swim, rinse and comb a conditioner through your hair. Your hair acts like a sponge and there's only so much water it can adsorb, so the wetter it is before you go in, the less chlorine it will absorb.

The sun, saltwater and chlorine will suck the moisture out of even the healthiest hair. Drink plenty of water to keep your body well hydrated. As well as keeping your body healthy, remember that what you put into your body will have a direct impact on your hair.

Wash your hair less often. Washing hair strips out natural oils and moisture, which the hair needs when in regular contact with the sun's rays.

Give your hair a summer makeover. Get a trim to remove damaged ends so your hair will be stronger and more manageable during the summer months. And don't forget to go every 4-6 weeks to keep your hair in optimum health.

Reduce the amount of heat generating styling methods, such as blow drying and straighteners. If you do use them, use a leave in conditioner and/or a good heat protection product.

Don't use very hot water when washing your hair, this is another way that your hair can get dried out and damaged. Use warm or cool water instead.

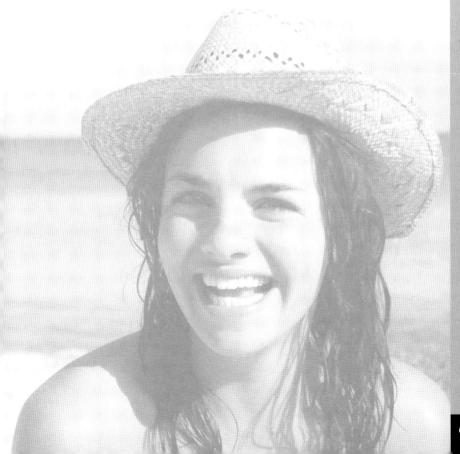

Hair Myths exposed

Cutting your hair makes it stronger or grow faster.
Cutting your hair will only make it shorter and hairs grows about half an inch per month. Cutting your hair regularly will ensure that it remains it good condition and can therefore appear stronger.

Brushing your hair is good for it.
Acutally over brushing your hair can be bad for your hair and is a leading contributor to split ends and hair breakage.

Washing your hair everyday dries it out.
Once you have found the right shampoo for your hair type and texture, washing every day can actually add moisture and body.

Hair can turn grey or white over night.
Hair receives its colour genetically and can only turn grey or white over very long periods of time. Hair doesn't actually turn white, rather it loses colour, but this is a lengthy process, not visible to the naked eye until the process is complete.

If you pull out one grey hair, two will grow back.
When you pluck out a grey hair all you are doing is removing dead tissue. Removal of the dead hair cells does not cause faster growth or thicker hair. In fact, hair cells turn off and on periodically-if you pluck a hair out, new hair may grow right away or not, depending where in its cycle the hair cell at the bottom of the follicle is in at the time. But the new hair will not necessarily be grey - but it is a fact that once you have found your first grey hair there is no turning back!

Our bodies are all wonderfully unique and come in all different shapes and sizes. When you look in the mirror do you know what shape you are and how to dress to compliment your best bits? Want to make more of your wardrobe, improve your clothes-shopping expertise and get some great fashion tips? Look no further! Try these easy to follow fashion tips for a more stylish, confident, fashion-savvy you.

Fashion tips and body type

This useful guide will help you figure out your body shape and what's best for you – a great tool for choosing your clothes and feeling more comfortable and self-assured in what you wear.

Hourglass

This shape has bust and hips in proportion with each other, with a well defined waistline. Pretty much the shape of a literal hourglass. A great shape for many styles of clothing, but beware of drawing too much attention to curvy hips, if you're uncomfortable with them, by defining your small waistline too much. Cropped jackets and fitted waistcoats look fantastic, as do tops that don't cling to the waist area.

Hourglass curves should be shown off so don't them hide away underneath baggy clothes.

If your hips aren't an issue for you corsets and pencil skirts are a fantastic way to accentuate the waist area.

Sophia Loren is the archetypical hourglass figure, with Halle Berry and Scarlett Johansson typifying today's hourglass figure.

Athletic

This is an ideal shape for just about anything that you want to wear. But don't become a fashion victim by trying to wear every fashion trend. Celebrities with athletic figures include Cameron Diaz and Keira Knightly.

Pear-shaped

Pear-shaped bodies have wider hips than shoulders, so the aim is to balance out proportions. Clothes ideal for this shape are empire line dresses, straight legged trousers, A-line skirts and tops with low necklines accentuating your bust and drawing attention to your upper half. A bold print top and good accessories are also good for diverting attention away from the hip area.

To emphasise your bust area further go for halterneck tops and dresses, corset tops and tailored jackets. A strapless dress fitted down to the waist and flaring out in an A-line will look fabulous. Famous pear-shaped celebrities are Jennifer Lopez and Beyonce.

Apple-shaped

The opposite of the pear-shape, apple-shaped bodies are larger on the top and smaller below. This body shape usually has a short neck so elongate the neck by wearing v-neck tops. Avoid tight clothing around the upper body, anything that clings will draw unwanted attention to the waist area. Flared skirts and wide legged trousers are all great for this body shape.

Straight body

The straight body is proportioned the same from the bust area to hips, with no definition of the waist. To flatter this body shape wear clothes with dropped waists and accentuate other areas of the body, such as the legs, bottom and bust area. Avoid high clothes with high waists and belts, which will draw too much attention to the waist.

Soften your shape with necklines that draw attention and interest to your chest area and enhance your bottom with a dress with a flare, or a tulip-shaped skirt to pull in your waist and add needed volume to your hips.

Petite

Most retailers cater for petite sizes these days, taking away much of the nightmare of constant alterations. The right fit is naturally going to be paramount, but you don't have to stick in petite ranges if the standard fittings look just as good.

Wear darker colours as they will lengthen the body, as will skirts that finish just above the knee by maximising the leg length. Vertical stripes are slimming on everyone but especially advantageous for petite women who want to appear taller. Capri pants also achieve a taller look, elongating the calf and lengthening the leg. Shift dresses are good for creating balanced proportions for petites. Kylie Minogue typifies this body shape.

Big bust

You'll either love 'em or hate 'em – but if you want to minimise your top-half wear v-neck or scooped necklines, although not too low if you are self conscious about showing too much. High necklines will only serve to accentuate your top half and make you look even bigger. If your bust is attracting far too much attention, minimise them with an empire line that sits on your bustline. A good fitting bra is essential; a good bra will lift your bust and give definition to the waist. Balcony bras look great on bigger chests.

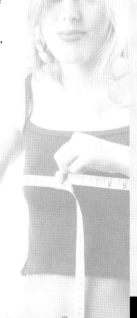

Small bust

Create a cleavage with 'chicken fillets' and consider wearing ruffles, or a smock top, to enhance the look. A bra with spaghetti straps will provide enough support.

Keep the bras pretty if your straps are going to be showing under strappy tops and dresses.

Big hips

To minimise attention to big hips wear wide legged trousers in dark colours, this will lengthen the legs and detract from the hips. Tailored clothes with a professional cut are excellent for flattering big hips.

Chunky arms and legs

If you're feeling conscious of flabby upper arms choose three-quarter length or half-length sleeves.

For bigger legs choose a skirt length which ends just above the slimmest part of your legs. For example, if you're unhappy with your calf area, don't go for a three-quarter length skirt. For big thighs but slim calves a knee-length skirt will give the appearance of slim legs all the way up.

If you don't like wearing shorts because of larger thighs, consider wearing long shorts. This will allow you to get your pins out whilst hiding the parts you don't want seen. Boot cut trousers are great for larger thighs as they make them appear slimmer.

Short legs

If you're not blessed with long, lean looking legs – or if you simply want to make your legs look longer – wear footwear with a heel, creating the appearance of thinner calves and longer legs. If you're uncomfortable with the height of stilettos then wear a smaller heel. Avoid shoes with ankle straps as these cut your legs off at the ankle, making them appear shorter.

Another fashion faux-pas are Capri pants, these cut your legs off at the ankle area, making your legs look shorter. This also doesn't help if you're not happy with your ankles, as this will accentuate them further. Opt for boot-cut style trousers instead, which streamline your legs and give them length.

Essential style basics

Quick and easy to remember style tips:-

Fashion victim

Don't become a fashion victim! Don't wear it just because it's in! There's nothing more ridiculous looking than someone wearing head-to-toe fashion regardless of style or suitability. Plus which, trends come in-and-out in a virtual heartbeat and will cost any fashion devotee an absolute fortune – remember, what's hot will soon be NOT!

Class act

Keep it classy. Show off your breasts OR your legs, never both in one outfit unless it's on the beach.

Age wise

Dress age appropriately. If you suspect that a style looks too young for you, trust your instincts, you're probably right!

Asset management!

Learn to recognise your best assets. Know your body and which are your best bits. Choose clothes to flatter and accentuate the positive.

Pale fabrics

Be careful of wearing white, pale or pastel shades in cheap fabrics as they can look rather unflattering and emphasise parts of you that you'd possibly rather keep under wraps.

Well-fitting clothes

Wear clothes that fit well and don't either drown or strain across you. Tight clothes especially will make you look bigger than you are, not to mention showing every slight bulge and bump.

Colour control

Watch colour contrasts. If you're of a heavy or petite build avoid dramatic contrasts between your top and bottom half. The contrast will cut you in half and make you look shorter and stockier.

Skin deep

Sallow skin or dark circles. Avoid wearing black near your face as this will only highlight the problem.

Common sense

Good hair, nails and skin. It won't matter what stylish masterpiece you're wearing if the rest of you looks unkempt and shabby! A good hairstyle, polished nails and glowing skin will set off your outfit and make you look and feel fabulous.

Natural beauty

Keep an element of natural beauty in your look, you can't go wrong.

Dress yourself slimmer!

Basic style tips to dress yourself thinner:-

Enhance and highlight your great bits! If you have killer-legs, draw attention to them in a stylish mini, or if you have a slender neck optimise your look with tasteful jewellery and accessories. Drawing attention to your good bits will also detract attention away from the bits you want to hide.

If you're conscious about your width, stay well away from horizontal stripes. They widen your shape and make you look bigger than you are. If you like the striped look, opt for thin, vertical stripes instead as these will flatter your torso and make you look longer and thinner.

Poor posture can add pounds to your look, so stand up straight, hold your head high, pull in your tummy and hold your shoulders back! It's amazing what a difference your posture can make, not only to how your body looks, but also to how you feel. An upright, self-assured posture looks fabulous and exudes confidence – as well as slimming you down in seconds.

Wear clothes that fit! If you wear ill-fitting clothes you WILL look bigger – either because your clothes are unforgivingly tight, or because you're swamped by excess material. Many people hide under layers of fabric and shapeless clothes to hide weight issues, but this will only make you look bigger. Buy well-fitting, good quality clothes and you'll instantly look better.

Make sure you have the right support, i.e. good underwear. If you have no issues with body fat, or any lumps or bumps, then underwear can be as skimpy as you like. But if you're trying to 'hold in' certain body areas, good supportive underwear is a must – pulling in the tummy, buttocks or thighs and providing lift to your bust.

Don't wear heavy fabrics, they will make you look bigger. Choose finer, silkier materials.

Buy clothes which skim over the areas of your body you want to detract from and disguise. For example, if you have a tummy bulge stay away from tight, clingy tops and opt instead for a tunic style, or empire line top;

this will skim the stomach and make it appear flat. However, be careful not to buy baggy items, as these will automatically make you look bigger.

Don't buy cheap clothes. If you have a fuller figure you will need good fabrics and quality cuts to compliment your shape. So don't be duped into a cheaper wardrobe with lots of styles and fabrics that don't quite fit or hang right. Instead invest in your wardrobe and buy a few well-chosen classic lines that will suit your figure.

If you have thicker ankles, avoid delicate, strappy heels, ballerina-style shoes or ankle straps which cut across the ankle, making them look bigger.

For bigger arms choose bell-shaped sleeves to cover up.

Black – the essential for every wardrobe. Black clothes are well known for their slimming appearance and can be easily accessorised for an evening look. But remember that a proper fit is still your principal priority.

Learn what colours suit you and inject them into your wardrobe. Bright coloured clothes are fine to wear, again as long as they suit your colouring and fit properly.

Don't wear shiny or glittery fabrics, which will draw maximum attention over parts of your body that you might want to minimise.

Don't be a fashion victim. Rule of thumb for any shape or size, don't buy something because it's 'in-vogue', buy clothes that suit and flatter you individually. If you're a fashion devotee and 'must have' the latest fashions, dedicate your energies into the latest accessories which will compliment your wardrobe.

Heels are your new best friend! Wear high heels to elongate your legs and calves.

Don't ever wear tight clothing – no matter what your well-intentioned skinny friends say!

Accessories

Tips for those all-important accessory items that will work to enhance and improve your look. Use your accessories to create maximum impact:-

Stiff leather and junky-style shoes and handbags will cheapen your style; quality goods will enhance and give you a classic look.

Never wear black shoes with bright colours as they will make your outfit look cheap.

If you have a rounder face or double chin go for longer earrings. These will elongate your face and chin.

If you have a short neck don't wear choker-style necklaces or scarves with your outfit.

Don't buy monogram bags, especially if they're from a secondary line. Fashion fads apply to bags too – best to keep your label inside the bag!

If you have a bigger bust avoid wearing long necklaces and pendants that end in your cleavage. This will draw too much attention to the area, for the wrong reasons!

Roll-neck jumpers should be left plain – never wear a necklace or scarf over the top.

Don't wear your pashmina wrapped tightly around you like a coat, it's meant to be draped elegantly around you.

Good quality, well-fitted underwear is a must. Your gorgeous outfits won't look right without the necessary support and figure enhancing undergarments.

Get a great look, which will slim you down and draw attention to your impeccable taste by investing in a good quality, big bag!

Have fun with your handbags – choose some lively colours and different shapes. An old-fashioned handbag can unwittingly add years to your look.

Avoid ageing yourself prematurely and don't wear overdone, fussy styles with too much detail. Opt for unfussy chic: minimalist designs and details.

Belts shouldn't make you look bigger. If you want to slim down your look, wear a belt with a slight diagonal slant, wearing the buckle at the side to detract attention away from your tummy. If you want to emphasise a small waist then wear a high-waisted belt to pull you in and accentuate your curves.

Don't wear tights that show through your toenail polish (i.e. sheer tights). Yuk!

Don't buy printed tights with patterns; unless you're aged 7 or under!

Don't overdo the glitz and 'bling-bling'. The right amount of shiny accessories can look great, but avoid looking like you wouldn't be out of place in Harrods Christmas scene window!

If you're constantly battling with time and have no space to commit to a lengthy beauty regime, this may be just what you need. These 5-minute beauty shortcuts are great for a busy lifestyle, optimising precious spare time whilst making you look and feel a million dollars.

5-Minute morning routine

Avoid morning mayhem with these easy to follow tips for looking your best.

Cleanse and moisturise

There are a myriad of products and recommended cleansing routines available. But if you're stretched for time, invest in a gentle cleansing bar or foaming cleanser, and indulge in an old-fashioned wash with warm water.

There are plenty of soaps and foaming cleansers formulated to be kinder to skin and respect your skin's natural acidity.

This is a quick, easy and less messy alternative to creams and lotions. They're also easy to rinse off and a final splash of cold water will bring colour to your cheeks, firm your skin and act as a refreshing 'wake-up'.

Massage in your usual brand of moisturiser to hydrate and soften your skin.

Cheeks

A hint of colour on the cheeks gives your face a healthy glow first thing in the morning.

Smile in the mirror and apply your blush to the apple of your cheek, sweeping it back towards the cartilage nub in your ear. Applied too low blusher will make your face look wider.

Eyes

Our eyes are the first thing that people notice about us, and this is certainly true first thing in the morning when we're regaining wakefulness after a full night's sleep.

Once you've washed and moisturised, a light coating of mascara on the upper lashes will open the eye up and make you look more awake.

There are great lengthening products on the market if you want to achieve a longer, fuller lash look.

Lips

In the morning, using a slightly damp toothbrush, very lightly scrub your lips to remove any dry flakes.

This will also stimulate the circulation giving you rosy, warm looking lips.

Add a little lip salve to moisten your lips.

Hair

For mid to long hair, if you're pressed for time you can just pull it back into a ponytail or with clips. Use a non-stick hairspray to tame fly-away hair.

Scent

To finish off, use a body spray or a little perfume. Something light and fresh, you don't want to overpower anyone!

Skin

It's rare that we can get up, look at our skin and be completely happy with what we see in front of us.

Most of us have something that we want to cover up or disguise, whether it be blemishes, spots, broken capillaries or dark circles. Rather than cover the whole of your face with foundation, just touch up any areas of concern with a foundation that best suits your skin tone.

If you're in a particular rush, you could try mixing your moisturiser with your foundation – saving you having to put on two products. Either that or invest in a tinted moisturiser.

5-Minute make-up tips

Tips for times when you have only minutes to get a great look and get out the door:-

 Apply an all-in-one foundation and powder product; this will give your skin the right amount of coverage – and in half the time.

 Buy 2-in-1 products that can be applied on cheeks and lips, or cheeks and eyes. These keep your colour tones similar and save time.

 For a quick, effective eye opener, apply a shiny highlighter below the arch of the brow and in the inner corner of the eyelid. This will open and lift the eye.

 Cream eye shadow applied straight from stick is quick, easy and stays on.

 One coat of mascara is enough for top and bottom lashes. Invest in good quality, ophthalmic approved mascara for optimum looks.

 Using a brow pencil, define your eyebrows to give your face more definition and impact.

 A touch of powder blush can be applied using a big blusher brush for a fast, effective look. Sweep up from your cheek towards your eyes.

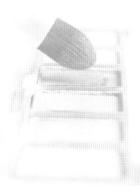 To create the illusion of a slimmer face use bronzers and highlighters. Sweep some bronzer under your cheekbones and apply a highlighter above your cheekbones, then blend together.

For a healthy glowing look dust some bronzer onto your brow bone, nose and chin.

Use a neutral colour or translucent lipstick for a faster application and a natural look. Less precision is needed and no lip-liner.

Shaking off any excess, dab a translucent powder with a velour puff over your face to prevent shine and finish off your make-up.

Use disposable make-up remover wipes for removing eye shadow and mascara. Baby wipes are just as good!

5 Minute Beauty Tips

5-Minute essential basics

Tips essential to our everyday beauty routine:-

Cleanser

Dermatologists recommend that a gentle cleanser is the most effective way to cleanse your face. So if you're a die-hard scrubbing with soap and water person then you may want to revise your thinking. Over-washing or vigorous washing can strip away the skin's natural barriers and moisture.

Washing with a gentle cleansing product no more than twice a day is the kindest way to cleanse your skin.

Have the right beauty tools

There's not much point in spending a small fortune on the best beauty products but not investing in the right tools to apply them with! Any large department store will stock full ranges of beauty tools and brush sets.

Lips

How many of us take our lip-care for granted? They're one of the most sensual features on our faces, and one that comes into regular contact with other people! Considering their high-profile function we don't spend nearly enough time looking after our lips and enhancing their natural beauty.

The number one rule for lips is to keep them hydrated and moist. Prevent dry and cracked lips with lip balm, use a balm with an added SPF when outside. Use lip balm during the day and before you go to bed at night.

For a gentle, natural looking pout apply a little petroleum jelly to your lips and rub it in. Follow with lip balm.

Moisturise

If you have time for nothing else in your daily routine, prioritise time to moisturise. The type and brand of moisturiser will depend upon your skin type, individual needs and preferences, but never underestimate the importance of moisturising. Moisturisers plump up and smooth the skin and protect us, to some degree, from premature ageing. Start using moisturisers young and reap the benefits in later years.

Sunscreen

Most of us know that sunscreens help reduce the risk of skin cancer, but they are also a vital beauty ingredient in keeping our skin looking young. The sun adversely affects the amount of collagen production in the skin, which is essential in maintaining plump, moist, youthful skin.

Not only does sun damage cause more wrinkles and fine lines, but also more freckles, age spots, and spider veins. Skin can also start to look rough and leathery, or loose and saggy because of sun exposure.

Sunscreen with an SPF of 15 or over can protect skin from the sun's damaging rays, so that even if you spend time outdoors your face is less likely to suffer sun damage and add unnecessary years to your age.

5 Minute Beauty Tips

5-Minute facial workouts

A non-invasive way to help to firm up skin, maintain good circulation and achieve a radiant, youthful look to your face and complexion:-

Double-chin buster

Sit at a table and, with a closed, relaxed mouth jut your chin forward and slightly upwards. Rest one elbow on the table and clench your fist. Balance your chin on your clenched fist. Slide your lower lip out and over your top lip. Press the tip of your tongue against the roof of your mouth behind your top teeth. Increase the pressure over a count of 5 hold the position. Slowly release the pressure. Repeat the sequence 3 times.

Forehead firmer

Raise your muscles above your eyebrows and gently but firmly use your fingers to smooth out the forehead wrinkles. Repeat the sequence 3 times before raising and dropping your eyebrows quickly 20 times.

Lip conditioner

Imagine you're playing to a room full of adoring fans and blow 10 kisses in quick succession. Then repeat by pressing two fingers lightly against your lips and blowing 10 more kisses. A really fun way to firm lips!

Firm droopy eyelids

Look straight ahead and place your index finger lengthwise just under your eyebrows. Keeping your eyes open, gently push up your eyebrows and hold them firmly against the bone. Slowly close your eyes and feel the pull between brow and lashes. Squeeze your eyes tightly together and hold for 5 seconds. Release the pressure over another count of 5. Repeat the sequence 3 times.

Jaw and neckline workout

Jut your chin upward so that you can feel that the front of your neck is taut. Push your lower lip over your top lip towards your nose. Keeping your neck stretched, slowly smile by pulling the corners of your mouth upward and outward over a count of 5 seconds. Hold this position for another count of 5 and firmly stroke the jaw-line upwards with the flats of your hands. Release the position slowly over a count of 5. Repeat the sequence 3 times.

Super fast tips to achieve super looks:-

 Test new foundations on your cheek not on your hands. Our hands are darker on the back and paler on the inside.

 Don't have time for a tan? Invest in some bronzing powder for your face and shoulders.

 Use neutral shades and you won't have to worry about your cosmetics clashing with your clothing.

 Lip colours – the deeper or brighter the colour the more obvious it will be when it starts to fade. If you don't have time to re-apply endlessly stick to a safer, more subtle tone.

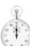 Periodically sharpen all of your make-up pencils so you're not fishing for the sharpener at the last minute.

 For blobbed and clogged mascara use a clean, damp mascara wand to separate out the clogged lashes, and a damp cotton bud to clean blobs up from the surrounding area.

 Add a finishing touch to your lips with lip-gloss, giving you the appearance of plumper, more luscious looking lips. Keep it in your handbag for touch ups!

 Foundation sunk into your skin creases? Use a cotton bud to clean out and re-blend.

 Overdone the eye shadow? Blend a tiny dot of concealer on the centre of your lids to calm the colour.

 The skin on your chest will show signs of ageing just as much as your face and neck, don't neglect this zone and moisturise daily.

Bronzing powders make good blusher substitutes if needed. Choose the right bronzer according to your complexion.

 Strengthen weak and brittle nails by using a good nail hardener, (from salons or chemists). Massage oil into the nail base daily and moisturise well.

 Use an all-in-one shampoo and conditioner.

index

Index

Index

Index

Index

Superfood Recipe Index